Yes, Holistic Treatment and Development is Possible!

Learn How to Look beyond the Symptoms and Cure Your Entire Person

By: Sara Petterson

9781681275109

PUBLISHERS NOTES

Disclaimer – Speedy Publishing LLC

This publication is intended to provide helpful and informative material. It is not intended to diagnose, treat, cure, or prevent any health problem or condition, nor is intended to replace the advice of a physician. No action should be taken solely on the contents of this book. Always consult your physician or qualified health-care professional on any matters regarding your health and before adopting any suggestions in this book or drawing inferences from it.

The author and publisher specifically disclaim all responsibility for any liability, loss or risk, personal or otherwise, which is incurred as a consequence, directly or indirectly, from the use or application of any contents of this book.

Any and all product names referenced within this book are the trademarks of their respective owners. None of these owners have sponsored, authorized, endorsed, or approved this book.

Always read all information provided by the manufacturers' product labels before using their products. The author and publisher are not responsible for claims made by manufacturers.

This book was originally printed before 2014. This is an adapted reprint by Speedy Publishing LLC with newly updated content designed to help readers with much more accurate and timely information and data.

Speedy Publishing LLC

40 E Main Street, Newark, Delaware, 19711

Contact Us: 1-888-248-4521

Website: http://www.speedypublishing.co

REPRINTED Paperback Edition: 9781681275109:

Manufactured in the United States of America

DEDICATION

This book is dedicated to Floyd – my partner in life and in crime. Our marriage is the adventure I have always dreamed of. Thank you for keeping it real.

TABLE OF CONTENTS

Chapter 1 - The Role of Goal Setting in Holistic Development

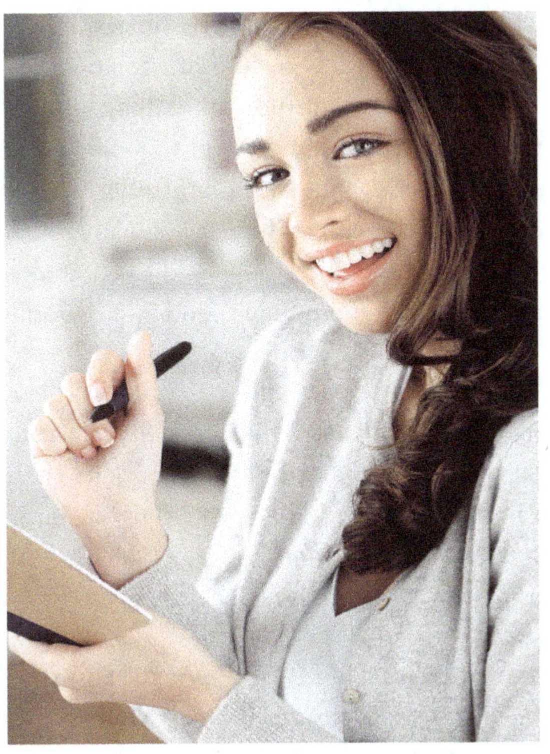

Right after your arrival in this world, you already have the destined thing to attain, which is your goal. Your goal in life depends upon your choice or preference. If you wish to be like someone you idolize, then so be it. If you want to gain a profession that is adored by most, you also can. But the thing is you need to properly set that particular goal in mind in order for you to attain it. Properly setting the goal you want to achieve will give you the chance to live a balanced life. In addition, the things you do in order to set and attain this goal will reflect who you really are. If you get to set them in the right track, then you can be close to achieving your holistic growth. Hence, it is important to use the best strategies that will guide you to accurately setting your goal.

Goals Are Meant To Be Set

Humans are destined to live a complicated life. This is seen right after the first time you opened your eyes to see how complicated the world could be. Living this unsure life could sometimes make each individual feel like giving up rather than asking the logical question "why live if it is meant for you to suffer and die?" Life is full of extreme difficulties, but these difficulties are the ones that make life worth living. Each creature living in this world has their individual goals and aims, which they need to complete in order to make the most of every minute they spend in this world.

However, not all individuals are sure of what goal they really have in life. Are they born just to live their life without having anything they want to attain? Or are they born to experience how boring life could be? A boring life is possible if you allow it. But, if you have something in mind that you want to attain, which is your goal, then you can say that living your life is never boring.

However, having a goal alone is not enough. You should think of what you can do in order to attain it. Goals can never be truly called goals if they aren't being acted upon, but if you just set it and you don't do anything to achieve it, then that goal is unsound. On the other hand, properly setting your goal is highly important. This could be your first step to accomplish it. Knowing how to properly set your goal is associated with holistic growth.

Why Holistic Growth?

"If you wish to achieve worthwhile things in your personal and career life, you must become a worthwhile person in your own self-development"- Brian Tracy

Wanting to achieve valuable things will in turn require you to be a valuable person in your own growth or personal development. This is what is meant by Brian Tracy in this quotation. Being a full-grown individual is an advantageous phase of a person's life. Once you say that you are full-grown, it will be easier for you to set your goal and then eventually attain it.

Have you ever wondered why there are lots of individuals who try reaching their goals but end up unsatisfied? Well, it is quite obvious – they have not matured enough to set their goal and at the same time, they are uncertain of what it will take for them to feel satisfied. This is where holistic growth takes place.

It is definitely hard to define a mature individual or to identify if he/she really has achieved holistic growth. Holistic growth can be achieved when you include all the necessary things surrounding the concept. Say for example, when it comes to an individual with holistic growth, then he/she must have a balanced mechanism. This mechanism includes his/her physical, emotional, mental aspects and the like. Once these major aspects are properly balanced, then you can tell that the person has achieved holistic growth.

However, if you will link holistic growth to goal setting, it may be simple. Since holistic growth for a person should involve his vital aspects, as mentioned earlier, for goal setting it works in the same manner. Putting it simply in a sample situation, say for instance, you are a server from a certain restaurant and what you serve there is twice as much as what you usually eat on a regular basis. For some reason, you made a goal of eating the whole meal.

However, if you make it as your goal, you are probably not considering your holistic self. If you are thinking holistically, you'll certainly not set such a goal because other aspects of yourself may be given a negative effect. Say for example your health, if you consume too much, then you may have high levels of cholesterol, which can lead you to unwanted illness. Hence, it becomes highly important for you to consider each and every factor that will be affected by the decision you will make. Be mature enough to consider each factor.

Chapter 2- Basics of Holistic Growth Setting

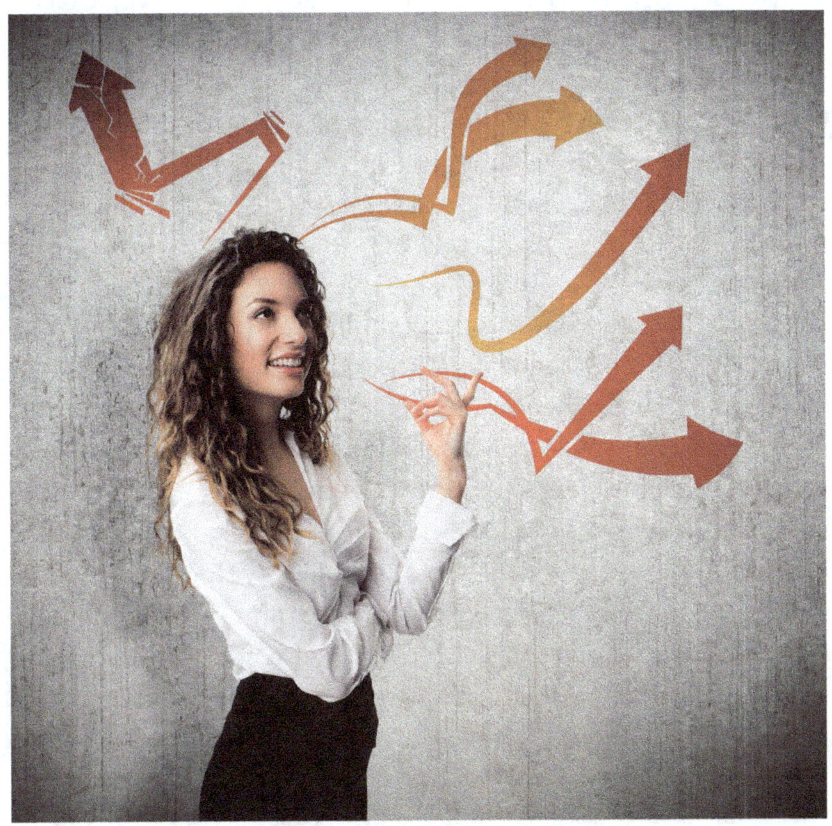

Your task does not only surround goal setting. For example, you have set your goal already, but you don't really know if that goal you set is enough at that. Doing this thing is never holistic. You should be very careful right from the very start of setting your goal up. This is important because who knows if that goal is missing something crucial. Then you may be at risk of not attaining it.

Therefore, it is important to understand goal setting principles. What are these principles, and how can they help you become successful in attaining your goal? Well, continue on to find out.

The Principles

Goal setting basically includes the seven crucial principles. These principles include the first one, which is specifying what you exactly want. If you are certain about your goal, then it can be easier for you to reach it without struggling so much. The second principle is about the practicality and attainability of your goal. Be sure that the goal you are trying to achieve is not impossible. This is important because in time you will be the only one who will benefit from it.

The third principle focuses on your desire to attain your goal. Your desire should be high enough, which can be used as your personal motivation. Think of the possible things that may happen if that goal is already in your hand. Visualizing and living with your goal is the focus of the fourth principle. This is in connection with imagining your desire. Imagine how great it could be if your goal has already been attained is a helpful way for you to stay motivated about reaching your goal. The fifth one is listing or writing down your goal. This principle can also help you from being successful in attaining their goals based on a number of studies.

The sixth principle involves the time allotment you are giving to your goal. This is also very important because it will help you to keep reminded about your goal. Make sure to include the time frame in your notes, so as not to forget about it. The last, but not the least, goal setting principle is taking the goal into action. Once, you already learn the principles that need to be understood, it is then the time for you to start running to reach the finish line, which is your goal.

There are times when people find it quite hard to set their goal because of too much confusion. Things can be worse if you have a number of goals, which you may not be able to think what is good to do with them.

Set Your Goals Using the Principles as Your Guide

The first principle you need to know and apply is to clearly specify your goal or what you desire. As mentioned earlier, the goal needs to be specific and clear. In order to arrive at the right place, you first need to exactly where you are heading. The second principle is that your goal needs to be attainable and realistic. Do not set a goal that is impossible. A situation for this is dreaming about winning in a lottery without even first buying a ticket, or aiming to have a million dollar without doing anything besides imagining it. These kinds of instances actually happen in reality. You should be true to yourself. Yes, it is free to dream, but if you really are determined to reach a particular goal, then set one that is achievable and not the one that is obviously unattainable. Therefore, after you specified your goal make sure that it is realistic.

The third principle in goal setting involves your burning desire. Make sure that you have a high desire for that goal in order to attain it. One factor that can help you get this desire is to become highly motivated. You may think of the great things you can experience once that particular goal becomes successful. Think that nobody can stop you from reaching that goal, so it will be easier for you to get it in no time. HOWEVER, always remember to be holistic at all times. As mentioned earlier, you should always consider that the things on the way to reaching your goal should never be left negatively affected.

The forth one is to imagine and live with your goal. When you identify your goal, try to imagine all the factors and envision yourself living with it as frequent as possible. Visualizing is extremely important because it has powerful effects. Be inspired by the inspirational quotation stated by Napoleon Hill "What the mind can conceive, and believe, the mind can achieve". Therefore, you need to make sure that you spend some time visualizing and focusing as if your goal is already taking place.

The fifth one is to list your goals. Studies have shown that the goals that are written on a paper are much more effective than those that are merely thought of. These studies have also shown that the ones who take note of their goals have achieved even more as compared to the ones who didn't write down their goals. Therefore, you may want to get in the habit of writing down your goals, so as to monitor your goals and keep track of their progress.

Another step you should take is to identify your time frame for the goals. You always need to identify the time you want to complete your goal. Doing this will surely give you better motivation factor to attain your goal. In addition to this, just like the first principle you also need to be realistic of your time frame, consider if it is attainable or not, or if it fits your capability to finish it within the given time allotment.

The last step, but certainly not the least, is to act based on your set goals. Once you have done all the mentioned steps, it is then the time for you to execute your action to attain your goals. The first step is often hard, yet once you have done it, you will probably become familiar with it. Therefore, learn to take your first step without any doubt or delay to get success closer and closer to you.

Sara Petterson
The Benefits of Setting Goals

Setting your goal has a great deal of benefits. However, always think that having your goals properly set is important in order to achieve these benefits.

Make the Most of Goal Setting

Goal setting has a considerable number of benefits from which you will surely feel satisfied with. One of the benefits of goal setting is that it makes you feel conscious about your weaknesses, allowing you to enhance them by converting them into strengths. This is one evident and useful benefit of goal setting. Another benefit you can acquire from goal setting is that it provides you the sense of previous successes of accomplished goals, using them as your inspiration to become successful in your present goals. This one will probably give you an idea that having one goal at a time is much better than striving for them at once.

Goal setting can also assist you in visualizing and planning the necessary actions in order to attain what you desire through executing them. Setting your goal provides you the right track to run on, or the direction to follow, helping you become aware of the path you are going to. Setting your goals properly can give you more even more benefits by encouraging you to lay down your priorities, which probably limits you from participating in some distracting things or factors. This will then lead you to have a definite precedence to prioritize. Establishing your goals can also help you provide proper definitions about real life acts that separate them from fancy thinking.

Another crucial benefit that comes from goal setting is that it allows you to become responsible for your own failures and successes. Once you set your goals, you should be aware of the possible consequences when they fail, so it allows you to respond positively to them. This is the act of a responsible person. You should know and understand that not all the times success is for you, hence you should accept it once it's done. However, you should not stop from trying because setting goals is always there to help you. You can reset your goals into a better and more possible format, which will allow you to reach your goal this time.

Setting your own goals is also training yourself with purpose and intensity. Since striving for success requires burning motivation, it lets you become trained with intensity. This will enable you to be a tougher and stronger individual in return. Once you have a set goal, it also lets you identify and keep track of your goal's progress, making it more useful to you. You set your goals in order to enhance your mental and physical performance because of the things you typically encounter along the way toward reaching success. Having your goals properly set assist you in planning your time, balancing the many aspects of your life, keeping track of your achievements and assisting you in managing your everyday life.

CHAPTER 3- CAN YOU LIVE A BALANCED LIFE?

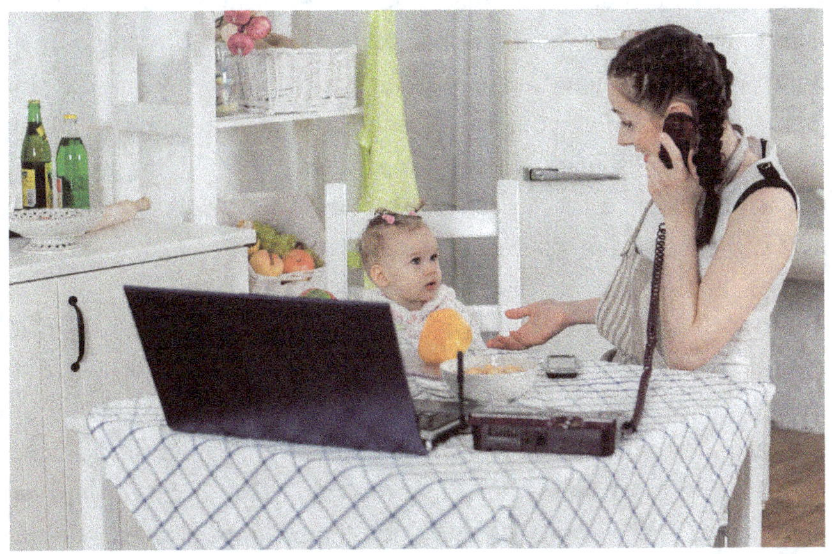

Setting your personal goal will probably lead you to have a better and a balanced life. How? Well, after you have identified what you want to attain in the various areas of your life, it is important for you to examine and observe how they go together. By doing this, you will surely realize how you come up with a balanced life through properly setting your goal.

Goal Setting to Live a Balanced Life

If you consider growing as an individual, there are several different areas you may think about. These areas probably include your desire to be a parent or spouse, growing in your social relationships, or perhaps in your career or job. Improving your mental and physical health, spiritual life and intellectual pursuits may also be included in these goals. Furthermore, you may also improve in your hobbies for enjoyment, or in your participation in the community.

Say for example you want to be a better parent. But then, if your personal goals and career requires you to be distant from your home for long, or allow you to be very busy in order to work well when you're at home, you may want to reconsider your priorities and then make some adjustments on your balance. This could be a great way to help you be clear about your values as well. You can create a list including your values and then accurately match them to your goals' list. See if they properly match or if there is any unbalance. If there is, you can make some adjustments, which will lead you to have a much better and balanced life.

Another thing that can help you attain a balanced life is to figure out what is most essential to your life. If you know and hold the most important thing in your life, then it will be easier for you to live your life to the fullest while living it in balance. In order for you to know the most important thing for you, it is helpful for you to understand the reasons behind their importance. Decide if you want to dedicate energy, time and attention to those things. Ultimately, you should decide if the goals you set will help you to become a well-balanced person, as being one will eventually lead to living a balanced life. Hence, these things make goal setting crucial to living a balanced life.

Goals and Balancing Your Life

Your goal is the particular success that you desire to achieve. In order to attain this goal, you should monitor it every now and then, allowing you to observe its progress. Progress occurs little by little. Your goal should be achieved within a specific time frame. This makes monitoring your goal really important. An exerted effort is vital in order for you to achieve the goal you set.

However, what exactly is the impact of goal setting to have a balanced life? What makes it beneficial?

Sara Petterson
The Real Impact of Goal Setting to Life

Goal setting has lots of benefits associated to it, which certainly includes giving you the chance to live a balanced life. Many people choose to set their personal goals in order to establish accurate direction. Indeed, this is very evident. Having a direction of what you really want to attain is what goal setting is all about. If you don't set your goals accurately, you will probably end up taking a zigzag path which will be very uncertain. On the other hand, if you have an accurate goal that you are viewing on the horizon, it will be easier for you to head to its path.

Goal setting has a strong impact on having a balanced life, which is one of its benefits. Setting your goals balances all the things that take place in your life. Say for example, your goal is to be a good parent who wants to guide his/her kids along by giving them positive and favorable thoughts. However, your job doesn't allow you to complete this goal. What is the right thing to do? Well, one of the most effective things to do is to adjust your schedule. It will be better if you will do what your heart and mind wants, so as to let you live a balanced life. Knowing that you have what you want is a great way to live your life in balance.

Setting goals, in addition, helps you live a balanced life because it motivates you to take action. If you haven't set your goals, how will you be motivated to act on it? Well, it may be, but at most times having the goals set is the major factor that helps people work harder. An example of this is when you wake up in the morning and go to your work. Will you consider waking up early if you know that you don't have any work to go to? People by nature are lazy at times; hence setting goals is one that helps them become motivated to try hard, striving to live a balanced life.

Another reason that makes goal setting important is when you have a certain goal is that it helps you overcome obstacles. You will carefully think whether a certain action you will make will affect the goal you are striving for or not. This will help you have a balanced life because there will be no further confusion that will take place in your mind.

The Intimate Relationship of Goal Setting and Success

Success is something that everyone wants to attain, but not all are given a chance to get hold of it. But then, even if this is the case, still people should not give up on attaining their goals. One of the common reasons why people fail in attaining the success they desire is when they don't get to properly set their goals; resulting in them feeling disappointed and sometimes even stressed out. There are ways you can avoid this. And first on the list is you need to know that success and goal setting are interconnected, and that none of them should be left behind.

If you want to gain success, the first thing you should do is to set your goals. Dreaming of success is useless if you don't set your goal for it, and of course perform the action. Goal setting is an extremely important ingredient you should know and understand in depth. Consider that you don't just set your goals to gain success, but you also do it to have a balanced life. Sometimes having a balanced life can be considered as one of the successes achieved from goal setting. You can consider it as success because it provides you peace of mind, without having to think about the confusions often encountered in life.

Keep in mind that success can never be attained without first setting goals. Therefore, to have a successful and balanced life, always choose to set your goals, in line with the things you want in life.

Chapter 4- Holistic Health Remedies that Work

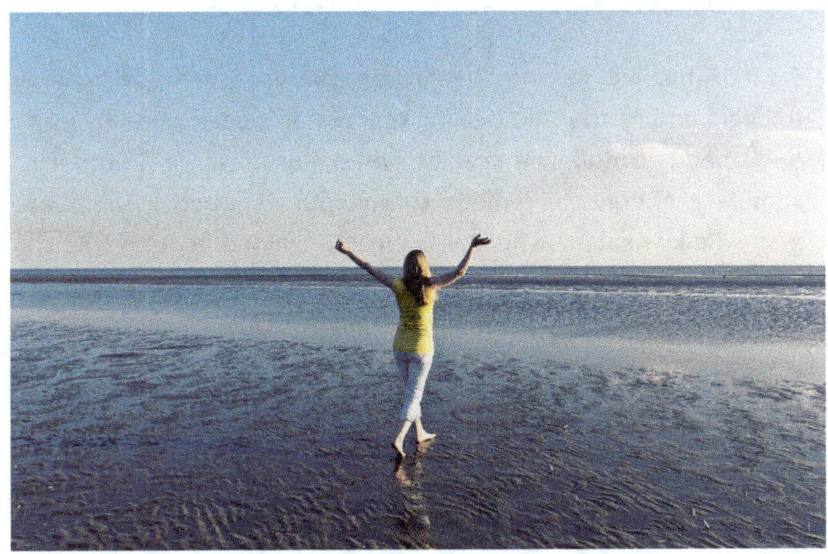

1. Improve your posture. It is important to keep your spine as straight as possible, so that your muscles do not strain and contract unnecessarily. Also, in order to keep energy circulating throughout your body, it is important to keep your spine straight and nerves unhindered.

2. Consider "trigger point massage" for pain relief. If you are plagued by continuous pain and conventional pain medicines are not working to help eliminate it, consider this special type of massage. It will help to not only ease the pain – but to eliminate its source as well.

3. Try acupuncture. Acupuncture is type of holistic/alternative medicine that has been commonly practiced in the eastern part of the world for thousands of years. Five thousand years ago, the intention of acupuncture was to prolong life. With many alternative medical techniques, the intention is to prevent rather

than to cure a specific or general ailment. The oldest recorded practice of acupuncture was over 5,000 years ago. Basically, acupuncture is used to stimulate the nerves in the body and as a result positively affect all of the other bodily systems.

4. Try Reiki healing. Reiki is a healing art that uses the body's energy to begin and further the healing process. It is performed by using one's hands to follow a specific pattern of massage, in order to stimulate energy movement throughout the body. There are many Reiki healers who are specially trained to perform the healing massage, or you can read about it or take a class to become a proficient Reiki healer yourself.

5. Consider a complete body cleansing. There are many different products on the market today that can help you to eliminate toxins from the body and increase the efficiency and overall health of your body. A complete cleanse will remove toxins and other harmful matter from your kidneys, liver and intestines. Generally how they work is you follow a strict dietary regimen for a few weeks while the cleansing process occurs. Most people who try this agree that it makes them feel healthier and they often report a fair amount of weight loss after the process is complete.

6. Try to avoid television. Believe it or not, television actually induces negative feelings in most viewers as a result of the commonplace violence and gossip. Television viewing is not nearly as relaxing as some people claim. Try giving up your television shows for a week, replacing them with other activities. You will most likely find that you are better rested, happier and less stressed at the end of that week.

7. Consider biofeedback therapy. If you are experiencing health problems and cannot seem to find the source, a biofeedback

therapist will monitor your body and how it reacts to daily activities in order to find out where it is not performing optimally. In this treatment, you would wear a monitor that actually records how your body is reacting while it is turned on. If you are an athlete suffering from muscle problems, you might want to consider this treatment to determine whether you are properly resting your muscles between activities.

8. Improve your sleeping habits. One of the best things that everyone can do to improve their well-being is to moderate their sleeping patterns. Unfortunately, poor sleep is a habit learned by nearly everyone during the teenage years. It is critical to allow your body the time it needs to wind down and relax so that you can be rejuvenated. If you feel tired during the day, when you awaken in the morning or exhausted before bedtime it is a sign that you are not getting the right amount of sleep. This could be too much, or too little. Try setting aside eight hours for sleep each night, getting into bed no less than half an hour prior to the time that you want to be asleep. If you do this for a few weeks, you will find positive improvements in your overall health and productivity.

9. Breathe mindfully. The process of mindful breathing is a form of meditation; however it is also a great way to get more oxygen into your blood and tissues. If you start right now and pay attention to how you are breathing, it is more than likely that you will find yourself breathing quite shallowly. This is not a healthy breathing pattern. You can start out by just inhaling completely and then slowly exhaling completely. If you take one minute to just do this focused breathing each day, you will find that you feel better during that minute. And, you will catch yourself paying attention to your breathing several times throughout the day. If you are stressed or tired, take a minute out of your day to breathe mindfully.

10. Meditate for better wellbeing. The basic definition of meditation is to concentrate on some object or thought in order to quiet the mind. There are many different types and styles of meditation; however the one thing that is consistent is that not every technique will work for every person. Everyone can benefit from some type of meditation, take some time to read about different techniques or talk to a holistic healer for more information about what might work for you.

11. Go to the dentist. If you have fillings that could possibly contain Mercury, it is a good idea to have those fillings replaced by your dentist. If you are feeling poorly and cannot explain why, this may be the culprit. Mercury poisoning is slow and often masks itself with symptoms of other health problems. Your dentist can tell you whether you should consider having any of your fillings replaced.

12. Consider a peroxide bath. Hydrogen peroxide is known for being a highly effective astringent that removes toxins, or dirt, from scrapes and cuts. It can do the same thing for the rest of the body as well. Simply add a quart of peroxide to your hot bath and soak for a few minutes to check for tolerance. If you don't have any irritation that does not stop quickly, add a second quart and soak for about ten minutes. The peroxide will pull toxins from your skin and help you to flush toxins better afterwards.

13. Consider a liver flush. Gallstones form in the bile ducts and the gallbladder, and may be to blame for medical problems that go otherwise unexplained. By performing a liver flush you are helping your body to eliminate the built up toxins and gallstones. If you are interested in instructions for a liver flush, you can find them at any reputable holistic healer and even online. If you have any health problems, or suspect that you might, you should speak with your doctor prior to performing the process.

14.   Consider learning from an Alexander technique instructor. The Alexander method is a way to retrain the body to remain correctly postured in order to prevent and eliminate the possibility of problems such as muscle strains, nerve damage, stiff necks and many more. The purpose of this technique is to eliminate unnecessary tension within the body and to teach the body to position itself correctly.

15.   Eat clay. Yes, clay in its naturally occurring form is fantastic for treating many different health ailments that might go otherwise untreated. Liquid clay is available and can be taken several times a day to help with problems with the liver, headaches, and arthritis and skin disorders. Clay masks are fantastic for the skin, and when used after a good exfoliation they can remove impurities and toxins from your skin.

16.   Consider "transpersonal therapy". If you have found that standard therapy is not working out for you, this is an approach that helps many people to feel more comfortable. In this type of psychotherapy, the therapist and the patient focus on making a significant connection with one another in order to remove anyone from a superior position. Many patients have found that when they feel a connection with their therapist, they feel that they can be more open-minded and receptive.

17.   Pay attention to your dreams. Dreams can tell you a lot of information that you might not otherwise realize. Therapists believe that through our dreams, we become aware of personal struggles, fears and internal conflicts. Consider keeping a dream journal, where you record at least the major themes of what you are dreaming. Do this as soon as you can after waking, so that you make sure to get the essence of your dreams. Pay attention to patterns, serial dreams and symbols that seem to reappear often. Find out what these things represent to you by meditating

on the symbol or theme, or look them up in a dream dictionary for the generally accepted explanation. While this may not represent the meaning for you, it will give you a place to start.

18.   Try yoga to overcome depression. If you are suffering from depression, practicing yoga may help you to overcome the symptoms and get to the root of what is causing the problem in the first place. Through the practice of yoga, you are attempting to connect to your spirit and to reconnect your mind and body. With practice, you may begin to see the symptoms of depression begin to lessen almost immediately.

19.   Consider color therapy. Try changing the colors in your wardrobe to better suit your emotional needs during any particular time in your life. For example, if you feel that you are in need of a personal change, or that you need to build your self-esteem, consider wearing purple, as this color is known for its connection with self-healing. If you are stressed, try wearing light blue. Green is a great color to add when you feel like you have recently made a personal accomplishment, since it is a color known for renewing effects.

20.   Try magnets for pain relief. Magnetic therapy is becoming a very popular method for treating chronic pain and conditions that cause chronic pain. Magnets are shown to increase blood flow through the body by as much as a third. This increased circulation is a great way to alleviate pain.

21.   Try bioenergenic therapy when you are feeling depressed or tired. Bioenergetics is an alternative therapy that includes a combination of different techniques used together to help your body fight off illnesses, depression and other conditions. Practitioners observe the patient and form a treatment plan that works to correct things like breathing patterns and stress levels in

order to begin identifying and alleviating problems that the patient is experiencing. This therapy combines biofeedback with talk and touch therapy, acupuncture and nutritional counseling in a specific way determined by each individual patient.

22.	Consider a whole body detoxification program. The environment, stress and even the foods that we eat can affect every cell in the human body negatively. Sometimes, the body just needs a break so that it can effectively remove harmful chemicals and byproducts that reduce the body's ability to fight disease and to function at its peak. A whole body cleanse will give you the ability to remove toxins from your intestine, organs and even your skin. Consider working with a holistic physician to see if a detoxification program could help you.

23.	Try what ails you to relieve the symptoms. Homeopathic medicine practitioners believe that a symptom is little more than the body's defense against stress. Therefore, they take the approach that finding a substance that behaves in the same way that the body does – that substance can be used to fight off the ailment or infection. Take a walk through a health food, or nutritional supplement store, and you are bound to see a homeopathic remedy for many common health problems.

24.	Try a natural caffeine detox. If you have been promising to give up coffee, or to cut down, you might need to actually remove the effects of caffeine from your system with a detoxification process that includes chamomile. This extract helps to calm you while washing caffeine from your system. You can use chamomile tea, or a specially developed compound designed to detoxify the body.

25.	Consider chiropractic medicine. If you are currently experiencing back pain, chances are that the damage has already been done. Chiropractors are specially trained to manipulate the body in a way that frees nerves and muscles to function correctly, thereby reducing pain in the body immediately. It is important to work with a Doctor of Chiropractic, who has attended college and Chiropractic College.

26.   Consider working with a holistic athletic trainer. If you are an athlete, you might benefit from the experience of working with a holistic trainer who focuses not only on injury recovery, but also on performance analysis, counseling and injury prevention. Through the holistic approach, your mental and physical needs will be addressed and you can improve your performance significantly as a result.

27.   Try Kinesiology to improve your wellbeing. Kinesiology is a holistic approach to traditional biofeedback therapy, where the body is studied in order to determine the source of potential and current problems. Through monitoring of your body, your Kinesiologist will determine a course of alternative treatments that will help you to perform to the best of your capabilities.

28.   Try hypnosis. There are many different schools of hypnotherapy, however all center on the idea of using altered states of consciousness to help you find and resolve issues within yourself. The primary goal of hypnosis is to be a short-term therapeutic process that can help the patient to find a deep issue that they have been unable to realize in their conscious mind so that they can begin to find a solution to the problems that they are facing.

29.   Try a homeopathic approach to ADD. ADD is becoming one of the most commonly issued diagnoses among young children and adolescents today. Unfortunately, the treatment options are limited and most include the use of strong medications with

terrible side effects. A better approach might be to treat only the symptoms that are present, and to treat in order to prevent the appearance of new symptoms. Homeopathic treatment includes not only natural medicines, but psychological counseling as well. The goal is to treat the patient, and not the disease. There are many traditional physicians who will work with you to develop a homeopathic treatment plan, and many holistic physicians who specialize in this type of treatment.

30.   Get real allergy relief. If you suffer from allergies, you already know the frustration of treatments that just don't work. Sure, they may mask symptoms for a while. But, they are not going to provide lasting relief. Homeopathic allergy treatment is different because instead of treating the symptoms, the goal is to strengthen the body to a point where it can resist the allergens that are behind the symptoms. While there are treatments available for the symptoms, a patient can expect to be given medications that make their immune system build upon itself to create a natural defense.

31.   Listen to more music. Sound therapy is becoming commonplace in homes with newborn infants and older adults. There are many benefits of sound therapy including calming and increasing the patients sense over overall wellbeing. Find a soft music that you enjoy, and try playing it at the lowest possible volume in a quiet room. You will find that before too long, if you are quiet and relaxed, that you hear the music as though it were at full volume.

32.   Become familiar with aromatherapy. Aromatherapy is a simple way to change your daily life. Through the use of essential oils, it is possible to get access to wonderful therapeutic results. Aromatherapy has been a popular holistic health topic for thousands of years, and many people will tell you that the

promised benefits are completely accurate. For example, consider placing a few drops of Rosemary oil on a cotton ball and dabbing it on your forehead during a headache. Or, consider placing a drop of lavender oil on the light bulbs in your bedroom for enhanced relaxation during sleep. Consult a pharmacist, holistic specialist or a book on essential oils to determine if one or more could help you to improve your well-being.

33. Eliminate the cause of health problems before trying to treat the symptoms. So, for example if you are suffering from indigestion it makes more sense to eliminate the foods that are causing the problem than it does to take medication after the pain starts. Holistic healers are looking to heal the whole body, and therefore it is believed that first you stop doing the things that are harming you, and then you replace those things with nutrients, etc. that are better for you. This can apply to the body, the mind or the soul.

CHAPTER 5- A NOTE ON HERBS AND VITAMINS

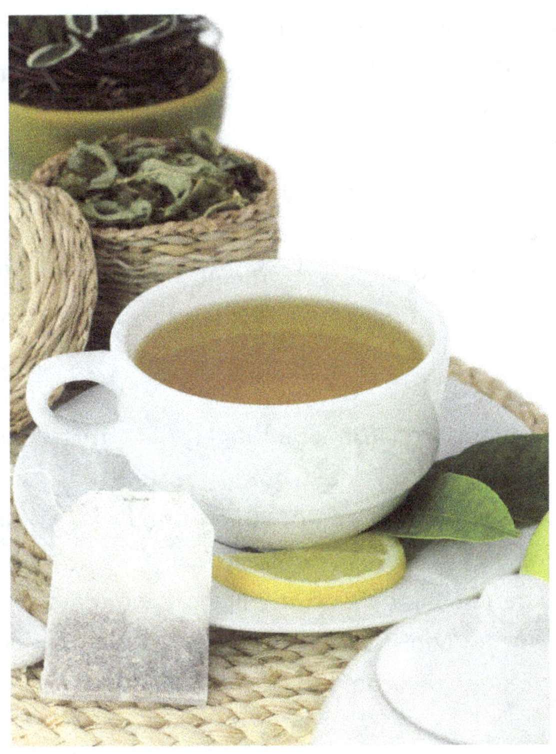

1. Get more vitamin D. Supplements are one way to increase your Vitamin D intake, however quite honestly the best way to get this nutrient is from sunshine. The human body synthesizes Vitamin D that is absorbed through the skin when exposed to sunlight. Many people are not getting the sun exposure that they require because of the risk of skin cancer; however in moderation – about 5 minutes a day - sunlight is very beneficial.

2. Take vitamin C prior to sun exposure. Getting sunburn is definitely unpleasant. By taking an extra dose of vitamin C prior to beginning your sun exposure, you are boosting your skin's natural defenses. If you would like increased protection, consider adding vitamin E as well.

3. Sooth your stomach with oranges and fennel seed. Make a mixture of a tablespoon each of orange peel and fennel seed added to two cups of water. Boil and then steep this tea. Add honey to sweeten the tea and drink it when you are suffering from indigestion. The tea should refrigerate for about 48 hours, and will taste primarily like fennel.

4. Drink rosemary tea. Rosemary is a kitchen herb known for its ability to stimulate the senses. If you are feeling tired, but have a lot to get accomplished you might do well to drink some Rosemary Tea. Rosemary Tea is also an excellent remedy for headaches.

5. Use ipecac syrup to stop vomiting. While this is one of the common ingredients in most home first aid kits, you may not realize that it is also a homeopathic remedy for vomiting when taken in very tiny doses. While ipecac will not do much for patients experiencing nausea, it will work wonders for you if you are experiencing continuous vomiting. A homeopathic physician or pharmacist can recommend exact dosages for you.

6. Take Ginkgo for better concentration. Gingko is known for its ability to stimulate the mind and to help the brain to metabolize nutrients correctly. In some cases, the herb has been noted to reduce the effects of aging and to slow the onset of Alzheimer's disease. Gingko leaves are ground into a powder and the extract can be used in many different forms. A few years ago, it became very common to see Gingko added to just about everything in the supermarket. A homeopathic physician can help you to determine whether you would benefit from a Gingko supplement.

7. Mix garlic and honey. If you are at risk for, or suffer from high blood pressure, consider eating a teaspoon of minced garlic

mixed with 2 teaspoons of honey every day. Honey and garlic are known for being healing foods, and when combined they are extremely beneficial to the circulatory system.

8. Soothe diaper rash with beeswax. Beeswax is the base for a homeopathic diaper cream solution. By adding in other herbs such as chickweed and marshmallow, you are creating a cream that is not only developed perfectly from nature – but one that will not stain and stick to your hands. This cream is far gentler than the conventional diaper rash creams currently on the market.

9. Try magnesium for leg cramps. Many people suffer from cramps in their legs, particularly in the calves. Drinking more water will probably help add magnesium to your diet is a great way to eliminate these cramps forever.

10. Try belladonna for ear pain. If you have an ear infection or ear pain, belladonna extract could possible help to alleviate this pain. This extract helps to reduce inflammation in the blood vessels, one of the common causes of ear pain. Other ailments for which belladonna will help include toothaches, fevers, restlessness or insomnia and eye pain resulting from dryness.

11. Take St. John's Wort for stress. This plant extract is known for its ability to help relieve the symptoms of depression, grief and anxiety. You can also try taking St. John's Wort for any injury that causes sharp pains or a repetitive stress injury. This supplement is commonly added to teas, and is also widely available in capsules and tablets.

12. Consider poison ivy for an ankle sprain. Although it is not commonly thought of as a good thing, poison ivy extract is actually an excellent pain reliever for sprains and strains.

Sometimes, the extract is given to patients with severe flu symptoms or even arthritis.

13.   Use chamomile for teething. Homeopathic remedies for teething contain this extract, which is known for its calming effects. The safest way to use this extract is in a cream or gel designed specifically for teething babies. There are specifically designed capsules that are placed under the baby's tongue to induce calmness and relieve pain.

14.   Use onions to relieve allergy symptoms. Onions are an excellent treatment option for those suffering from allergies because the root is completely natural and proves to be very effective at opening nasal passages. It's not as simple as eating an onion however. Because onions cause the same symptoms that allergy sufferer's dread, an extract should be taken in tiny doses, until the body begins to ignore the irritant and to develop a defense against the patients other allergens.

15.   Try lavender on your feet. If you suffer from athlete's foot, you already realize that there is little you seem to be able to do in order to stop the affliction. That is true with traditional medications. However, using oils of lavender, garlic and tea-tree in an alcohol solution will help to ward off the problem once and for all.

16.   Try peppermint oil for headaches. If you get chronic tension headaches and have found conventional medications to be failing, it might be a good idea to consider trying peppermint oil. A few drops of this oil can be placed on a cotton ball and applied to the forehead. Take a few minutes to relax and allow the oil to penetrate the skin.

17.   Sleep better with a sesame oil scalp massage. Warm a small amount of sesame oil, and massage into the scalp before washing your hair in order to induce sleep. This can also be an effective technique to stop a headache. Scalp massage in general is a good treatment option, however when combined with sesame oil the effects are better felt.

18.   Try Passion Flower extract. If you suffer from anxiety disorder, depression or hyperactivity this extract can help eliminate daily anxiety, calm hyperactivity and relieve stress. The calming effects of this extract are also thought to help with high blood pressure.

19.   Reduce stress naturally. One of the most commonly treated medical conditions in the world today is anxiety disorder. Thankfully, nature provided us with natural stress relievers like passion flower, lemon balm, lavender and valerian to name a few. Consider trying these various extracts to test their effect on your anxiety and stress levels with essential oils, teas and other forms.

20.   Try feverfew for headaches. Feverfew has been used for centuries by medical experts to treat rheumatoid arthritis and migraine headaches. This root is known for its ability to reduce swelling and fevers as well. You can try a tablet, or even a feverfew tea.

21.   Try vitamins C and B for a hangover. If you happen to overindulge with alcohol, you should immediately drink a glass of water and take some Vitamins B and C. This combination will start to remove the alcohol from your bloodstream and start the process of recovering so that you feel better faster.

22.	Try bee products for arthritis and joint pain. If you suffer from stiff joints or arthritis, consider trying bee venom in any of its popular forms. You might try a cream made from royal jelly, eating raw honey or even using bee venom itself. If you are interested in experiencing the healing relief of bee venom, contact an apitherapist, who will actually administer bee stings to your affected joints. If you are allergic to bee stings, you should not consider this treatment.

23.	Try ginger for joint problems. If you experience joint pain or stiffness, you might benefit from ginger caplets, or simply more ginger in your diet. Ginger is an antioxidant that is known to assist the body in preserving cartilage. You can find ginger supplements in any health food store.

24.	Try coriander oil for joint pain and stiffness. Coriander oil or extract can be added to mineral oil for massaging sore joints, or it can be brewed into a tea. Try making a 1 to 5 solution in an oil of your choice, letting it sit for 24 hours and then applying to sore joints.

25.	Stop sneezing with Echinacea. This herb has been used for thousands of years to treat the symptoms of the common cold. It is thought to be an excellent immunity booster. There are many different forms of Echinacea currently on the market. Depending on whether you are taking it as a preventative supplement or to treat current symptoms, the dosage may differ.

26.	Add more B to your diet. Foods rich in the B vitamins and B supplements are thought to be some of the most beneficial to the human body. B vitamins are excellent for the nervous system, the skin and are even used to treat respiratory problems including asthma. Foods like brown rice, baked potatoes and fish contain vitamin B. Try adding more to your diet today.

CHAPTER 6- CONSIDER NATURAL FOOD CHOICES

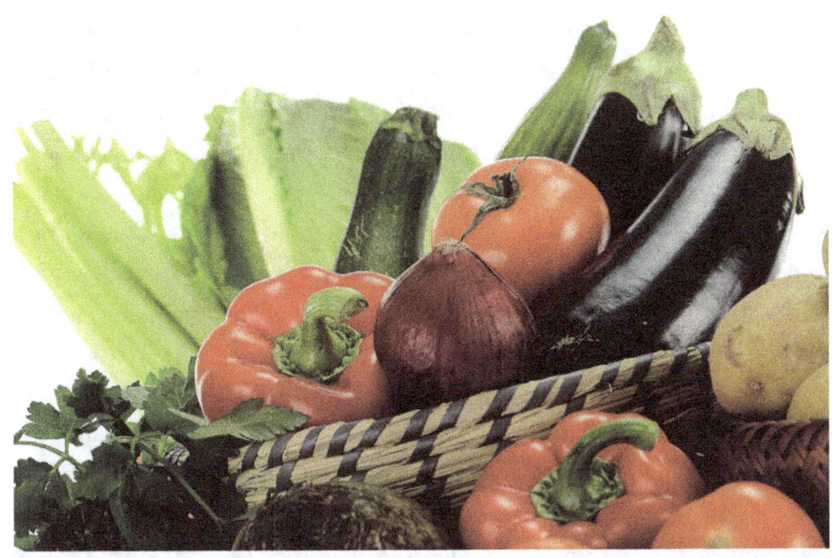

1. Improve your food choices. Many people who eat unhealthy diets believe that they are following a sound nutritional plan. However, those same people often do not include fruits and vegetables with every meal. And they often eat meals on the go without giving it a second thought. If you want your body to perform at high-efficiency, you must provide it with high-efficiency foods. This means more whole, raw foods and as few preservatives as possible.

2. Plan your eating ahead of time. This is one of the things that nutritionists will tell you to do when you want to improve your eating habits. For one thing, you will not be hungry if you are prepared with a meal schedule. Also, you will not be tempted by sugar and caffeine throughout the day when you have plenty of healthy alternatives on hand.

3. Drink more water. Most people cannot honestly say that they drink nearly enough water. In fact, many people do not realize

how much water they need to drink throughout the course of a day. You should focus on drinking half of your body weight in ounces each day. And, this does not include beverages other than water. In order for your body to function at its optimal, you need to make sure that you are drinking enough. Dehydration can occur when you are not getting enough water in your body, and there are many dangerous and bothersome side effects.

4. Eliminate the color white from your diet. In general, foods that are white in color contain little in terms of health benefits and are in fact better eliminated completely. This includes white bread, white pastas, potatoes, crackers that are not made from whole wheat and white rice. You can eliminate these items or replace with foods that have a higher nutritional value like whole wheat bread and pasta, sweet potatoes and brown rice.

5. Eat more foods that are acidic and alkaline. Consider modifying your diet to include foods that are acidic and alkaline, because many holistic experts believe that this is one of the keys to maintaining a healthy body. Foods like meat are high in acid. Fruits and vegetables tend to contain a high alkaline content. One of the reasons that this will improve your health is that your body will contain far less bacteria when it is acidic than when it is not.

6. Don't overdo the grains. Consider reducing the amount of grains and other carbohydrates that you are eating on a daily basis. The typical food pyramid emphasizes eating a large quantity of starches, however nutritionists believe that focusing more on fruits and vegetables will keep you healthier overall.

7. Consider adopting a raw food diet. This is where you eat only unprocessed and uncooked foods. Often, the damage done to the body by food occurs because of the additives and

preservatives that are used in the preparation. While most people find that they cannot sustain this type of diet for an extended time period, some have transformed their life and health through raw food consumption.

8. Avoid foods with added supplements. Believe it or not, nutritionists do not recommend supplements for the sake of adding more nutrients. You should try to obtain the nutrients you need through the foods that naturally contain them. And, if you require supplements, you are far better off just taking supplements. One nutrient that seems to be added to everything these days is calcium. The amount of calcium being added to products like orange juice is so minimal that it really will not help you to overcome a deficiency.

9. Eat a teaspoon of honey every day. Honey is known for its amazing healing properties, and because it contains 100% natural sugars it is a safe and effective way to give you an energy boost. Honey is good for your skin, your circulation and for the cells of your body due to a high content of antioxidants.

10. Nourish your body. Holistic healers believe that malnutrition is often responsible for many commonly occurring health problems, meaning that if the body does not get what it needs, illness will be the result. Imagine of you completely avoided calcium. The result would be brittle and broken bones and teeth. Well, the same applies for many other important nutrients. So, be sure to keep giving your body what it needs to stay healthy.

Holistic Approaches to Skin Remedies

1. Eat a better diet for better skin. Holistic specialists who deal with dermatological problems will tell you that most skin problems

are related to the foods you eat and the quality and amount of nutrients that you ingest. They will most likely point at food based toxins that seem to be keeping your skin from functioning effectively. One possible treatment that might be suggested is liver detoxification, considering that the liver is responsible for filtering most toxins out of the body.

2. Drink more water for skin problems. If you are suffering from a skin problem such as acne, eczema or some other sort of condition, the answer may be as simple as drinking more water. Improperly hydrated bodies lead to skin that is not supple and nourished enough to stop these conditions and dehydration can definitely cause skin problems that might otherwise be avoided. Make sure to drink 8-10 glasses of water every day. Making the change will help your health to improve overall, and your skin will show the results.

3. Treat your skin with Jojoba oil. Jojoba oil, in its many forms is an excellent supplement for your skin and hair. This oil is known for rejuvenation of the skin as well as repairing hair and scalp problems. Consider using a shampoo or body wash that contains the oil in order to have healthier skin and hair beginning right away.

4. Do not use anything on your skin that you would not also eat. While you naturally are not going to eat soap, you should purchase products that contain natural substances and little in the way of toxins or potential irritants. Otherwise, you are requiring your skin to work harder to eliminate toxins.

5. Try sulfur for acne relief. If you suffer from teen or adult acne, it might be worth trying a sulfur based cream specially formulated to work on skin lesions. Sulfur is a naturally occurring substance in the body, and therefore it is completely safe. There are a

number of conditions that can be helped by sulfur, in addition to acne. These include liver damage, shortness of breath, pink eye and lactose intolerance.

CHAPTER 7- STEPHEN COVEY'S 7 HABITS FOR HOLISTIC PERSONAL DEVELOPMENT

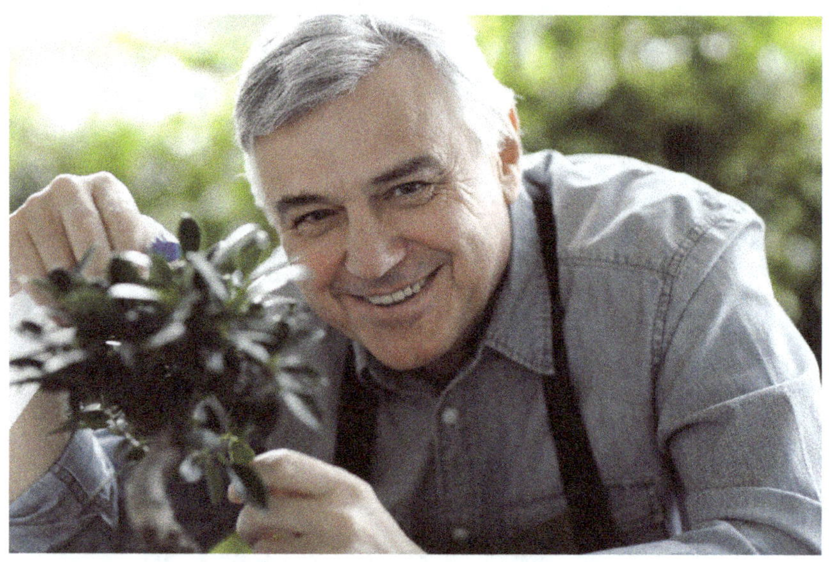

When Stephen Covey first released The Seven Habits of Highly Effective People, the book became an instant rage because people suddenly got up and took notice that their lives were headed off in the wrong direction; and more than that, they realized that there were so many simple things they could do in order to navigate their life correctly. This book was wonderful education for people, education in how to live life effectively and get closer to the ideal of being a 'success' in life.

But not everyone understands Stephen Covey's model fully well, or maybe there are some people who haven't read it yet. This is definitely true because we still see so much failure all around us. Now, I am not saying that by using Covey's model, or anyone else's model for that matter, you can become a sure-shot success, but at least we should have seen many more successes around us already judging by the number of copies the book has sold! So, where is the shortcoming?

There are two main problems here, and we are talking only about the people who have read the book already. The first problem is that most people are too lazy to implement the ideals of Stephen Covey in their lives. They consider his masterpiece of a book as a mere coffee-table book or a book that you use for light reading when you are traveling and then forget all about it. They do not realize that this book contains life-changing information. Or, they take the information and do not make the effort to actually utilize it so that it becomes knowledge for them.

The second problem is that a lot of people have a myopic view of Covey's ideals. These are people who are impressed by the book already. If you ask them what the seven habits are, they can rattle them off end to end, but then they miss the larger picture. They do not understand that Covey was trying to tell more than he wrote in words. There are hidden implications in this book, yes, and a lot of people have just failed to see through them.

That is what we are trying to do. We are trying to show you how Covey's book, or rather, his model, was a complete model in itself. There was nothing amiss about it. If you implement it, there should be no aspect of your life that should go untouched. The only thing is that you have to understand these ideals and try to implement them in your life.

But, before we barge into that area, it is extremely important to understand what these ideals are. What was the model that was propounded by Stephen Covey in his mega-famous book? We shall begin by trying to understand his model first, and then interpret it in such a way that it pertains to every aspect of our life.

Stephen Covey's Seven Habits

You must have read these habits in so many places by now. However, I do not mind repeating them for you here.

Habit 1: Be Proactive

Habit 2: Begin with the End in Mind

Habit 3: Put First Things First

Habit 4: Think Win-Win

Habit 5: Seek First to Understand, then to Be Understood

Habit 6: Synergize

Habit 7: Sharpen the Saw

Habit 1: Be Proactive

To be proactive, according to Covey, means that you have to be accountable to yourself. Your life is not perfect right now, however rich or poor you are. You always think that there is something lacking. A proactive person knows that something is lacking, but they do not start blaming external factors for those shortcomings. They won't blame their parents, their family professions, their country's economy, their lack of education, the weather, etc. Proactive people will raise above all this. They will understand what the situation is, they will realize that it can be bettered and that's that. They do not sit down and play the blame game, which is never anything but a gross waste of time.

Proactive people know that they can make their choices. They can choose to be happy or sad, they can choose to be pleasant or angry, they can choose to be complacent or responsive, they can choose to say yes or no. They have every choice. They are aware of this, and they take benefit of this fact.

A proactive person will never depend on others to make decisions for them. They will analyze the situation perfectly well and then they will decide what to do base on the merit of the situation.

Most importantly, proactive people are always optimistic. They are never shrouded in apprehension. They use sentences beginning with 'I can', 'We can', 'We should', etc. They do not think about the negative verbs. They do not thing that there is something beyond them. Even if there is something they have not achieved so far, they do not think that they are limited in doing so. If there is something they have not achieved yet, it is only because they haven't tried it. They always harbor the optimism that if they put an effort into it, they will definitely be able to achieve what they have set their minds to.

Proactive people are positive people. They are always sure of doing things, whether it relates to their family, their profession, their love life, their health, etc. They do not handicap themselves with limitations.

Now, that doesn't mean proactive people always meet with success. But this is only the first habit; we are just getting started. There are six more habits to go… it is only when all these habits are put in place in the right manner that things begin happening the way they should.

At the same time, you shouldn't get the idea that proactive people are obstinately optimistic. That isn't so. Practicality rules over everything. For instance, if there is a natural calamity or some other uncontrollable incident, then even proactive people may change their line of thought. This is acceptable. But, at least, proactive people will put in the attempt. And uncontrollable factors won't faze them. They will know that there is a way out… it is only about finding out what it is.

Habit 2: Begin with the End in Mind

Throughout history, we have observed that it is the farsighted people who have always achieved great successes. It is these people who have become legends and shaped the world in the way it is. Today, we see such people all around us. They are the people who begin with the end in mind. They are the people who are the diehard result-oriented people. They first think about what they want to do, what they want to achieve. The how's come later.

When you were young, you probably were asked many times, or maybe you thought about it yourself, as to what you would like to become when you grow up. This is actually a very common question and there are so many adults who ask it just for making a conversation with a kid. It becomes nice filler when you are talking to children. But, the next time you ask that to a child, listen and watch closely. Look at how serious the child is about what he or she says. They may say they want to become a fighter pilot or an astronaut or the next great legend in sports. But don't scoff it off with a laugh. Look at how earnest they are. Their eyes become totally expressive and there is some kind of a thought process going on in their little mind.

Now take yourself back to when you were a kid… when you were asked the same question. Perhaps you don't remember it now, but in all likelihood you answered the question in the same way. You have the same fervent zeal and appeal. You were totally earnest about your ambition too, even if it sounded ludicrous to everyone else.

Then, what happened on the way? Why did your aspirations falter? Did you, like most people, make some kind of compromise for some reason and put a tether on your galloping horse of imagination?

Covey tells us, in no minced words, that that is not the attribute of a highly effective person. If you have to be highly effective, then one of the most important things you have to do is to stay true to your ideals.

And that is what you can do by beginning with the end in mind. First, sit down and think what you have to achieve. This may not be something as mammoth in proportions as your life's ambition. It may be something small like a business goal. But, sit down and think. Think hard about wanting to achieve that whatever you are thinking about. You should think so hard that you should begin visualizing the success already. You should be able to taste your achievement!

When you are able to do that, you will find that automatically everything that you do falls into place. By already envisioning what you want to do, you have already set the wheels in motion. Consciously or subconsciously, you are working towards those ideals.

Most people have it pegged on all wrong. They start with the start. That's wrong. You have to start with the end. Think about the end. Whatever you are doing, your efforts... why are you doing them? What do you want to achieve at the end of the day? What is the end you are chasing?

When you start from that point, you know precisely what you have to do. Every waking—and even sleeping—moment of your life becomes a step in the right direction.

Habit 3: Put First Things First

We are humans and we are born and have to live with certain limitations. One of these main limitations is that we cannot do everything that we want to do. We have only a fixed capacity—a limit of doing things—and it is very difficult for us to go beyond that.

However, successful people have crossed these troubled waters. The more successful you are, the more things you will have to tackle. Successful people have managed to keep the boat going by focusing on only the most important things that need to be done at a particular moment.

Prioritization.

That is the game successful people play. They always see what's on their platter and then they pick and choose those things that absolutely need to be done. They know the art of prioritizing very well. And that is the reason why they are able to accomplish tasks. Maybe they do not accomplish everything... maybe they are not able to do everything that they want to do... but they are definitely able to do the most important things. They are able to do the things that can take them and their teams towards success.

But, how do you decide things that are the most important? What gives you the ability to do that? One way to decide your priorities is simply to see which of the tasks in front of you are the most beneficial, and I am not speaking only in terms of money here. See everything that is on your agenda. List things systematically. Then highlight the things that absolutely need to be done.

Another way to do that is to decide which thing is important for the success of another thing. If there is something you could do so that another task's fulfillment becomes simpler, then you should do that basic task first. This way, you set up a chain of events, and it becomes convenient for you to accomplish your various tasks.

There is another connotation to this habit as described by Covey. This is a simple connotation actually, but has a profound significance. This implication tells us that we should get everything ready when we are setting out to accomplish anything. That is putting first things first too. Instead of directly plunging headlong into trying to fulfill something, we should sit down and think what we can do to in order to make the task fulfillment simpler... what ingredients or raw materials would we need?

Getting those things in order first would be an ideal way to chase that particular goal fulfillment. Once again, that would make the task simpler. Moreover, this is definitely a form of prioritization.

Habit 4; Think Win-Win

We have been conditioned to think, by our parents, teachers and society in general, that life is all about winning. Now, that is not wrong in itself, but the approach that we have been taught is definitely wrong. We have been taught to win at someone else's expense. Or, we have been taught to understand that if we lose, someone else will win. This has become our natural thought process, and we rarely do think in any other way.

But, what Stephen Covey tells us to learn is that life is not about winning at the expense of someone else... or losing if someone else wins. This is not the way successes are carved. In the world of successful people, the success has been of everyone.

Think of the inventor of the telephone... or the radio... or the person who first landed on the moon... or the one who created Microsoft... what is the common element in all these people?

The common strand is that it is not just they who won. When the telephone was invented by Alexander Graham Bell, everyone used it. Communication improved immensely, all over the world. When Guglielmo Marconi invented the radio, the whole world rejoiced at the new avenue of entertainment that had opened up. When Neil Armstrong and Edwin Aldrin landed on the moon, it was a giant leap for the entire humankind. When William Gates developed Microsoft, it is not just Microsoft Corporation that became the richest commercial organization in the world, but it is all of us who witnessed and benefited from that revolutionary phenomenon.

Our lives have been shaped by these things... by these people who did not stop to think about their individual victories. They only thought about how they could take someone else ahead as well... how they could improve the world that they lived in.

Thinking about the world is a long shot, but you should at least think about the people who are close to you. To give you the right interpretation of Stephen Covey's model for highly effective people, the one thing that is important is that you should not aim for victory at someone else's expense. Instead, you should think about how you can collectively move towards victory. Success, in the present times, is about collaboration and not competition.

The Internet has made this possible. The Internet has shown us that victory doesn't belong to a single person. In fact, if it belongs to a single person, it feels inadequate. Victory is something we need to share collectively. We have to think of the win-win situation in which everyone is a winner, no one is a loser.

Habit 5: Seek First to Understand, and then Be Understood

Many self-help experts have spoken of the importance of communication. Surely, you have heard of several such methods as well. You have certainly heard how important it is to communicate with others if you want to make an effective impact on them and in general.

Nevertheless, what does communication mean to you? For many people, communication simply means talking. They have the impression that communication means speaking out their thoughts and opinions to others and giving advice.

However, that is the totally wrong meaning of communication. According to Stephen Covey's guidelines, if you think about communication in this manner as well, then you are bound to come up with great failure.

According to Covey, communication is just as much to listen as it is to speak. In fact, when you are talking, it becomes more important to listen to what others have to say. When you do that, you are amassing information and knowledge. This is where you understand what you have to do... what can be done... in order to solve a particular problem. This is what you need to do in order to attain your goals and be successful in society.

Remember that in conversation, listening is a method of input while talking is a method of output. If you want to enhance yourself, you should know that input is always better than output.

Yes, Holistic Treatment and Development is Possible!
That is what this habit speaks about. You have to pay attention to understanding the other person. You have to understand what they are trying to say. Only when you have fully achieved that, should you go ahead and make the other person understand that. In effect, you have to hear out the other person first, and then put forth your ideas.

The correct method is first to listen what people are telling you. Evaluate the information you get. Is it right or not? Are you agreeable to what they said or not? You have to think about it. You have to see whether you are convinced of what you heard. The next step is to advice, if you have something constructive to say. If you realize there is a problem and you have a suggestion for it, this is the time to feel free and proffer that suggestion. Lastly, you have to interpret how the other person reacts. You have to see what their response is, and don't pass any judgments about what it might be.

This is how effective conversation needs to be done. Conversing is a means, communication is the end. The best way to communicate is to converse by first listening and then speaking out.

Habit 6: Synergize

Synergizing is the most effective form of cooperation. This happens when you get together with people and then work in a constructive manner. You work in such a way that you pool in everyone's best skills and create a force that is beneficial for everyone. It is all about creative and constructive cooperation.

Look around you. The best people in the world—the richest people, the most successful people—have never been alone. They have their own coterie of people whom they're hobnobbing with; people who have brought them towards their accomplishment of goals.

Moreover, how are these people selected? They are most often handpicked by the successful people… they are people having different talents, talents that the successful people themselves are somewhat limited in.

These tie in with the first habit of being proactive. When we started out, we made no bones about the fact that everyone has their shortcomings. Even the most successful people in the world falter at some point. Being successful does not mean that you have to be perfect in everything. In fact, people who are really successful have just one main talent that they bank upon.

But, the world does not run on one talent alone. A person cannot reach the super zenith of success because they just have one amazing talent. This talent is on the fore, but in the background there are several other things working. A super rockstar has an amazing band to back them up. A hotshot politician has a whole cabinet of ministers to assist them. An Oscar-winning actor had the entire crew of the movie at their disposal. A writer had their inspiration and a good publisher to market their books in the right manner. A prizewinning athlete had a coach and several other people to help them out.

The thing that you have to take away from this is that success is not an individualistic thing. Even though we feel that some single person has achieved success, the fact is that there are many hands to support them… hands that have carried them to where they have reached.

This is what synergy is. Synergizing with people means to choose people to guide you and then collaborate with them in the best manner possible. The person who can collect the right talent is the one who goes places.

Now, every person is going to be different. You may need someone for their particular skill but you may not like the person. Or you may not like a particular habit in someone. But, should you let that come in the way? People who are aspiring to be highly effective should not think about these petty differences. They should look at the larger picture and carry on. This is what needs to be done, if you are looking for real success.

Habit 7: Sharpen the Saw

The saw here refers to the biggest gift that you have, without which you are nothing. And that is—your own body. You are only as good as your body is, as its health is, and that is the reason you have to sharpen the saw repeatedly, which means you have to be very cautious about what you are.

Covey does not just mean the physical aspect of the body; he means to say we have to enhance our physical bodies, but we must also look at the spiritual and meditative aspect of our bodies. In general, we have to make our body better. We need to look at various aspects of our life and keep sharpening it as well.

To sharpen the saw, you have to start by taking care of your health. Is there any bodily ailment that is keeping you from reaching the heights that you want to reach? If yes, then your first attempt should be to take care of them. Secondly, are there any emotional or mental problems that are threatening to sap your strength? Once again, these are things that you should take care of. If needed, you should renew and revitalize yourself using whatever means are available to you.

The most important thing is that you don't just have to be healthy from the outside, but you have to feel good within. You may probably want to invest time in some fruitful activities or a hobby that you appreciate or something else that recreates you. This is a great idea, because it makes you a new person from within, full of good cheer and camaraderie. This is what you need to succeed.

About the Author

Sara Petterson is a doctor of alternative medicine. She believes that pill and medicines should only be taken when absolutely necessary. In one of her seminars, she even referred to medicines and pills as added toxins that cure the symptoms but only quite the disease temporarily.

Sara is a strong advocate of natural remedies.

Her passion can be traced back to her parents' influence. Sara was born into a farm where the nearest hospital is 10 miles away. When she was sick, her mom and dad would give her herbs to make her feel better. Throughout her childhood, she has never been to the hospital. The wonderful experience with holistic medicine convinced her that others should try it too.